Natural Essential Oil Remedies & Recipes

Using Essential Oils in Everyday Living

By Wendy R Selvig

Certified Aromatherapist &

Certified Raindrop Tech Specialist

Contact: Info@theoilyacademy.com
The Oily Academy Podcast & Website: TheOilyAcademy.com
Get Young Living oils at YoungLiving.com. If you want Wendy to
be your customer service rep, use enroller #1062622.

DEDICATION

To my family, who supports me as I pursue natural health to help us live and function better. Thanks to Erik, Erik III, Caleb and Josiah. I love you all so much.

TABLE OF CONTENTS

Acknowledgements & Disclaimer

I am a Certified Aromatherapist and certified in the Raindrop Technique (an essential oil-based massage technique). I've also worked for a non-profit organization for 20 years as a natural health researcher. I love natural health!

I fully disclose that I am a Young Living Distributor and educator and originally wrote this book for my team. However, I am publishing this book from the perspective that anyone can use these recipes with any oils they have. I personally can only recommend Young Living oils because I know they are safe, distilled in surgical stainless steel, and have no aluminum toxicity like many oils do. Please take *great care* before you put oil on your skin or in your mouth to know that there is no aluminum or heavy metals present. It is a valid concern. If you are interested in learning about Young Living oils, please get in touch with me at **info@theoilyacademy.com**.

I also have a podcast with over 100 episodes called *The Oily Academy*, where I talk about oils and natural health. I have over 70,000 downloads as of the date of writing this book.

I am not a doctor, and the FDA approves nothing I say. The statements in this book have not been evaluated by the Food and Drug Administration. These products are not intended to diagnose, treat, cure or prevent any disease. Please do not take anything in this book as a diagnosis, treatment, or health claim. If you have questions about your health, please ask your doctor or naturopath. People react differently to substances, and what has worked for me may not work for you. Do your due diligence and talk to your doctor. Recognize that information changes as well (and evolves) and that the information in this book may be outdated down the road. I'm presenting what I know to be valid in 2023.

This information is provided to help you in your research. You are ultimately responsible for your health. I bear no responsibility for the improper use of and self-diagnosis and/or treatment using essential oils. If you suspect you suffer from clinical deficiencies or health problems, consult a licensed, qualified medical doctor.

Lastly, you must choose to use high-quality essential oils. If you don't, my recommendation is to decide not to use them at all. Unless you know your oils are distilled in surgical stainless steel, you are better not to use essential oils because there is a high percentage of oils in the industry that come from the perfume industry, where oils are distilled in vats made from metals like aluminum. Aluminum is dangerous for human and animal health.

It is also essential that your oils do not have anything added to them. Thinners are commonly added to oils to make them cheaper to produce and sell. Thinners are common toxins that make oils dangerous. There are no requirements on labels that make companies report if the oils have metal toxicity or thinners. Even oils that claim to be 100% something can have things added to them!

Have you ever bought a Mexican Vanilla that says it is 100% pure on the bottle? Usually, when you turn the bottle over and read the ingredients, more ingredients are listed. How can they do this?

What is meant (and often misunderstood) is that the vanilla is 100% pure, but they may have added other ingredients.

It is the same with essential oils. A label that says 100% pure Lavender means that the oil in the bottle is 100% pure. But the companies are not required to tell you if they put industry standard chemical thinners or used toxic metal distilleries.

After looking at many companies, I settled on Young Living Essential Oils as my company of choice. I won't spend time in this book trying to convince you to purchase their specific brand of oils, but I feel completely comfortable using them on my skin, internally, and in the air for my family.

Of course, if you are interested in oils from this company, you can make a purchase at YoungLiving.com. If you want to be on my team and have me help you with customer service and education, use enroller #1062622. But if not, the information in this book can be applied to whatever oil you use.

Please use great care when choosing your oils. Any old oil from a natural health grocery store isn't guaranteed to be safe. And this book's information assumes you are using clean, unadulterated essential oils.

Chapter 1

Introduction, Brief History, and Practical Application of Essential Oils

The Brief History of Essential Oils

Essential oils have been used for centuries to treat various health conditions and promote well-being. You can look seriously at essential oils for tried and true natural remedies. Plants have been distilled and historically used as medicines since at least 2000 BC.

Essential oils have also been used in traditional medicine practices such as Ayurveda and Traditional Chinese Medicine. The ancient Egyptians used essential oils for both medicinal and cosmetic purposes. They were also used in ancient Greece and Rome. Jars of Frankincense essential oils were found in King Tutt's tomb, which was still viable. Using essential oils is not a fad or something new. So, you can rest assured that your hippie grandma didn't discover them for the first time; the ancient Egyptians did.

During the Middle Ages, essential oils were used in Europe to treat various ailments. By the 19th century, essential oils had become widely used in the Western world. The current medical industry even used them until the 1950s when laws passed declared the pharmaceutical industry couldn't make a profit off a natural substance.

These natural remedies are extracted from various plants, herbs, and flowers. They can be used topically, aromatically, or internally (if labeled correctly) to provide multiple benefits.

The Science of Essential Oils

Until the 1950s, pharmaceutical companies sold essential oils as medicine. Then laws were implemented that said people couldn't profit from natural substances. This, unfortunately, put essential oils in competition with the pharmaceutical industry. Since the health industry and medical complex are for-profit, essential oils have stopped being promoted. They were even marketed against in some instances, and people were told they were "hokey," "voodoo," and "hippie" oils.

Many people ultimately bought the marketing strategies of the medical industry and struggle to believe anything natural could be good for you.

But your great-grandparents knew better. And thankfully, the upcoming generations get it as well. Essential oils are highly concentrated plant extracts containing various chemical compounds. These compounds are responsible for the therapeutic benefits of essential oils, and they can be extracted from plants using multiple methods, including steam distillation, cold pressing, and solvent extraction.

The chemical composition of essential oils can vary depending on the plant they are extracted from, and different oils have different therapeutic properties. For example, lavender oil is known for its calming and relaxing properties, while peppermint oil is known for its energizing and invigorating properties.

If you do a little research on Pubmed.gov and enter the names of essential oils (try *Boswellia* – also known as Indian frankincense), you'll find that scientists and doctors like to study the natural things that benefit us.

Then they take it apart and add things to make it patentable and profitable. I love that the healing constituents are inherently in the natural oils and typically don't have side effects. Why fix it if it isn't broken? Try natural and unadulterated oils for their incredible benefits.

Practical Application of Essential Oils
Essential oils can be used in various ways to promote health and well-being. Some standard methods of use include:

- Topical application: If the oil is distilled in surgical stainless steel and does not have aluminum toxicity or chemicals added, you can apply it to your skin. Can you imagine if you had skin cancer and put an oil on it with aluminum in it? You could potentially feed the cancer! Better off to not use oils at all than to do that. Make sure your oils are pure, and then you can add them directly to the skin, or if your skin is sensitive, essential oils can be diluted with a carrier oil (any fatty oil like coconut, avocado or sweet almond) and applied directly to the skin to support your body in its effort to maintain balance and healthy body systems.

- Aromatherapy: Essential oils can be diffused into the air using a diffuser or added to a bath to promote relaxation and reduce stress. The whole science of Aromatherapy is to breathe it in through the nose. When you inhale an essential oil, those tiny molecules (usually under 300 AMUs) go up the olfactory nerve and cross the blood-brain barrier. They get into your bloodstream and your brain simply by smelling them.

- <u>Internal use:</u> Some essential oils can be taken internally to support overall health and wellness. However, it is important only to use oils that are safe for internal use. I will only use essential oils that I know are safe. There is a reason why there are warnings on the internet and people are afraid to consume essential oils. Pure oils are health-supporting, but impure oils can cause great harm! I use Young Living oils for my body and family. Any of their oils in a white-label or marked for internal use can safely be used to take internally.

Chapter 2

Safety Considerations with Essential Oils

While essential oils can provide various health benefits, using them safely and responsibly is important.

Again, I can't stress enough the importance of determining if your oils are distilled in surgical stainless steel. Young Living Essential Oils distills in surgical stainless steel and doesn't add chemicals to their oils. They also make sure the plants are non-GMO and they don't use pesticides while they are growing. This is why I love using these oils so much.

Skin Sensitivity

Essential oils are made of tiny molecules that travel through your skin quickly. The faster they travel through the skin, the more friction they create, and heat and discomfort may be felt. There is a simple and fast way to remedy this if you feel discomfort anywhere after applying an oil. Add a carrier oil (which is a fatty seed oil) to the spot immediately to prevent discomfort. Fatty oil molecules are much larger than tiny essential oil molecules. They grab onto the little molecules and quickly slow the absorption rate, fixing the discomfort.

Be careful if you have an essential oil on your hands and need to use the restroom. If you wipe and get oils "down there," you may be in for a very uncomfortable few minutes! If that happens, wipe with some fatty oil like coconut oil – or use cooking oil in an emergency. Or, if you get essential oils in your eyes, wipe some fatty oil into your eyes and then use a washcloth to wipe it all out. You'll get relief quickly. Essential oils aren't damaging your skin if you feel discomfort, they are just traveling too fast through the layers. Carrier oils will stop the movement almost immediately and slow down the absorption rate so that you get relief.

Photosensitivity

Essential oils are excellent tools for supporting our physical, emotional, and spiritual health. However, it's important to be aware of the potential risks and precautions when using them, particularly regarding sun exposure.

Some essential oils can cause photosensitivity, making the skin more sensitive to the sun's UV rays. This can increase the risk of sunburn or skin damage. It's important to know which essential oils are photosensitive and to take proper precautions when using them.

Photosensitive essential oils include citrus oils such as bergamot, lemon, lime, grapefruit, and orange. Other oils that can cause photosensitivity include angelica root, cumin, rue, and some types of parsley. These oils contain chemical compounds called furocoumarins, which can react with UV light and cause skin damage. In all my years of using essential oils, bergamot usually causes the most problems. Be aware of any blends you use that might also have bergamot in them.

If you plan to use photosensitive oils topically, avoiding sun exposure for at least 12-24 hours after application is important. This includes avoiding tanning beds and other sources of UV light. Cover up with clothing or seek shade if you must go out in the sun. You can also use non-photosensitive oils to support your skin and avoid the risk of photosensitivity.

Here is a list of some common photosensitive essential oils:

1. Bergamot
2. Grapefruit
3. Lemon
4. Lime
5. Orange
6. Tangerine
7. Angelica
8. Cumin
9. Rue

It's important to note that this is not an exhaustive list and other essential oils may cause photosensitivity too. As always, it's important to research and use caution when using essential oils, especially if you plan to be exposed to the sun.

Here are some non-photosensitive essential oils that can support your skin. If you are spending a lot of time in the sun, use these instead:

1. Lavender - soothes and calms the skin, great for after-sun care.
2. Frankincense - supports healthy skin regeneration.
3. Helichrysum - great for supporting the healing of damaged skin.
4. Chamomile - soothing and gentle for sensitive skin.
5. Tea Tree - has immune system-supporting properties to support skin health.

When using essential oils, always dilute them properly in carrier oil before applying them to the skin. This helps to prevent skin irritation and sensitization. If you tend to have sensitive skin, or are concerned about how your skin will react, you can do a patch test before using a new essential oil single or blend to avoid an adverse reaction.

Babies and Small Children

Remember how concentrated essential oils are and how small children's bodies are compared to adults. The general rule of thumb with essential oils is that you only put them on the bottoms of the feet with children under two. This skin is less sensitive, but you still may want to dilute it with carrier oil. My favorite oils to use for children are:

Lavender – on the bottoms of the feet to calm and relax and help them quiet down for a nap or bedtime.
Raven™ – A Young Living blend for respiratory support. Put on the bottoms of the feet or the back (if they are older than two) to help with respiratory stress. Substitute with Eucalyptus if you don't have Raven™.
Lemon – An oil that stimulates the brain and supports happy moods.
Endoflex™ - An essential oil blend that supports happy and healthy hormones for all ages. (Spearmint is the key oil here).
Peppermint – This helps with concentration and stimulates the mind. Great for story time or when working on schoolwork.
Frankincense – This single is calming and emotionally grounding. I like to add this to the diffuser along with Lavender when my kids need to be quiet and focused. These oils are also great on the bottoms of feet to help support the immune system if you feel your kiddo may be coming down with something.
Thieves™ - This is a very famous blend that strongly supports the immune system. This is a powerful blend of Cinnamon, Clove, Eucalyptus, Lemon and Rosemary. This is the blend that convinced me that essential oils worked. My son had a 104.5 fever, and a friend gave me a bottle of Young Living's Thieves oil. I put it on the bottoms of his feet every hour on the first day of his illness – really hitting it hard. I took him to the doctor, and he confirmed it was Influenza type B. After putting

Thieves™ on his feet every hour, he woke up fine the next day! I love this oil!

Chapter Three

Simple Cleaning Recipes

Essential oils are not only helpful in improving health and skincare but can also be used to create effective and natural cleaning products. Avoiding toxic chemicals supports your immune system and overall health. Also, all those chemical cleaners have endocrine disrupters that mess with your hormones. Using essential oils as cleaners helps you to avoid messing up your hormones. Here are a few simple cleaning recipes using natural essential oils:

1. **All-Purpose Cleaner**

- 1/2 cup of distilled water

- 1/2 cup of white vinegar

- 10 drops of Lemon essential oil

- 10 drops of Thieves™ essential oil (alternately use Rosemary, Lemon, Clove, Cinnamon & Eucalyptus)

Mix the ingredients in a spray bottle and use it as an all-purpose cleaner for surfaces such as countertops, floors, and bathrooms.

2. Window Cleaner

- 1/4 cup of white vinegar

- 1/4 cup of rubbing alcohol

- 1/4 cup of distilled water

- 10 drops of peppermint essential oil

Mix the ingredients in a spray bottle and use as a window cleaner for a streak-free shine.

3. Air Freshener Spray

- 1/2 cup of distilled water

- 10 drops of lavender essential oil

- 10 drops of lemon essential oil

- 10 drops of peppermint essential oil

- 2 teaspoons of witch hazel to help the oils disperse.

Mix the ingredients in a spray bottle and use as an air freshener for a natural and refreshing scent.

4. Carpet Freshener

- 1/2 cup of baking soda

- 10-15 drops of your favorite essential oil

Mix the ingredients and sprinkle them onto the carpets. Let sit for 15-20 minutes before vacuuming up. This carpet freshener will help absorb odors and leave a fresh scent.

5. Veggie and Fruit Soak

- 3 cups water

- 2 cups distilled white vinegar

- 1/3 cup baking soda

- 5 drops of lemon essential oil

Put veggies and fruits in a large bowl and set them down in the kitchen sink. Sprinkle the baking soda over the produce, then add water, essential oil, and vinegar. Mix and soak for 20-30 minutes. *Note that Lemon oil has d-limonene properties making it ideal for dissolving synthetic coatings used by grocery stores on produce.*

6. Stainless Steel Cleaner for the Kitchen

- 8 oz Glass Spray Bottle

- 5 oz Water

- 3 oz Vodka

- 25 drops Thieves™ oil (or Lemon oil)

Combine ingredients in the spray bottle and spray and wipe down stainless-steel appliances in your kitchen.

Natural cleaning products made with essential oils can be effective and help reduce exposure to harsh chemicals found in traditional cleaning products. Ditch the toxic cleaners and go natural!

Chapter Four

Skincare Recipes

Essential oils have become increasingly popular in the skincare industry due to their potential to improve the appearance and health of skin. Here are a few simple skincare recipes using natural essential oils:

1. Anti-Aging Serum

- 1 tablespoon of carrier oil, such as almond or jojoba oil

- 5 drops of frankincense essential oil

- 2 drops of lavender essential oil

- 2 drops of myrrh

Mix the ingredients together and apply to the face before bed. This serum may help reduce the appearance of fine lines and wrinkles.

2. Acne Spot Support

- 1 drop of tea tree essential oil

- 1 drop of lavender essential oil

- 1 drop of lemon essential oil

- 1 teaspoon of carrier oil, such as almond or jojoba oil

Mix the ingredients together and apply directly to acne spots. These essential oils may help reduce redness and support the body's ability to overcome bacteria.

3. Soothing Face Mask

- 1 tablespoon of raw honey
- 1 tablespoon of plain yogurt
- 2 drops of chamomile essential oil
- 2 drops of lavender essential oil

Mix the ingredients together and apply to the face for 15-20 minutes before rinsing off. This mask may help soothe and moisturize the skin.

4. Refreshing Toner

- 1/4 cup of witch hazel
- 1/4 cup of distilled water
- 5 drops of peppermint essential oil

Mix the ingredients together and store in a spray bottle. This toner may help refresh and cool the skin.

5. Long Lashes Serum

- 5 drops lavender
- 3 drops cedarwood

Add to your bottle of mascara to help your lashes grow!

Chapter Five

Hair Care Recipes

Essential oils can create natural and nourishing hair care products. Cedarwood and Lavender are known for helping hair grow thicker. Other oils are known for bringing out the shine. Here are a few simple hair care recipes using natural essential oils:

1. **Nourishing Hair Mask**

- 2 tablespoons of coconut oil

- 2 tablespoons of honey

- 5 drops of rosemary essential oil

- 5 drops of lavender essential oil

Mix the ingredients and apply them to the hair, focusing on the ends. Let sit for 30 minutes before washing out with shampoo. This hair mask may help moisturize and strengthen the hair. Double this recipe for long hair.

2. **Dandruff GO-AWAY Hair Mask**

- 2 tablespoons of coconut oil

- 5 drops of tea tree essential oil

- 5 drops of peppermint essential oil

Mix the ingredients and apply them to the scalp. Let sit for 30 minutes before washing out with shampoo. This treatment may help reduce dandruff and soothe an itchy scalp.

3. **Hair Growth Serum**

- 2 tablespoons of Jojoba oil
- 5 drops of cedarwood essential oil
- 5 drops of lavender essential oil
- 5 drops of rosemary essential oil

Mix the ingredients and apply them to the scalp every night before bed. This serum may help promote hair growth and strengthen hair follicles.

4. **Shine-Boosting Rinse**

- 1/2 cup of apple cider vinegar
- 1/2 cup of distilled water
- 10 drops of lemon essential oil

Mix the ingredients as a final rinse after shampooing and conditioning. This rinse may help boost hair shine and remove build-up from styling products.

Using natural hair care products made with essential oils can help nourish and improve the health of hair without the use of harsh chemicals.

Chapter Six

Nail Care Recipes

Fingernails are not only a means of self-expression and aesthetics, but they also indicate one's overall health. Proper fingernail care involves maintaining the health of the nails and the surrounding skin. In this chapter, we'll explore the benefits of using essential oils for fingernail care and provide tips for keeping your nails healthy.

Tips for Fingernail Care

1. Keep your nails clean. Wash your hands regularly and clean under your nails with a soft brush. This will help prevent the build-up of dirt and bacteria that can cause infections.

2. Moisturize Your Nails. Nails and cuticles can become dry and brittle due to environmental factors such as frequent hand washing, exposure to water, and harsh chemicals. Applying moisturizer to your nails and cuticles can help prevent them from becoming dry and brittle. Natural oils such as coconut or jojoba oil can be used as moisturizers.

3. Trim your nails regularly. Trim your nails straight across and file the edges with a fine-grit nail file. Avoid using metal files as they can damage the nail bed.

4. Avoid biting your nails. Biting your nails can cause them to become weak and brittle. It can also introduce bacteria and germs into your mouth, which can cause infections.

5. Use strengthening nail polish. Many natural nail polishes contain ingredients like biotin and vitamin E to help strengthen your nails. These can be used to protect your nails from damage and promote healthy nail growth.

Using Essential Oils for Fingernail Care

Essential oils can support the health of your nails and cuticles. Here are some essential oils that can be used for fingernail care:

1. <u>Idaho Balsam Fir Essential Oil</u> - Idaho Balsam Fir essential oil has properties that can help prevent infections and promote healthy nail growth. Mix 2-3 drops of Idaho Balsam Fir essential oil with a carrier oil such as coconut or jojoba oil and massage into your nails and cuticles.

2. <u>Copaiba Essential Oil</u> - Copaiba essential oil has properties that can help relieve discomfort and support healthy inflammatory processes in the nail bed. Mix 2-3 drops of Copaiba essential oil with a carrier oil and massage into your nails and cuticles.

3. <u>Lavender Essential Oil</u> - Lavender essential oil has soothing properties that can help reduce stress and anxiety. It can also help promote healthy nail growth. Mix 2-3 drops of Lavender essential oil with a carrier oil and add to a hand or foot soak.

4. <u>Vetiver Essential</u> Oil - Vetiver essential oil has moisturizing properties that can help prevent dry and brittle nails. It can also help strengthen and nourish the nails. Mix 2-3 drops of Vetiver essential oil with a carrier oil and massage into your nails and cuticles.

5. <u>Helichrysum Essential Oil</u> - Helichrysum essential oil has healthy inflammatory process support and healing properties that can help repair damaged nails and cuticles. Mix 2-3 drops of Helichrysum essential oil with a carrier oil and massage into your nails and cuticles.

Fingernail care is an important aspect of overall health and well-being. Incorporating essential oils into your nail care routine promotes healthy nail growth, prevents infections, and keeps your nails looking great.

Remember to keep your nails clean, moisturize them regularly, trim them properly, avoid biting them, and use strengthening nail polish. Use the essential oils discussed in this chapter to help support the health of your nails.

Chapter Seven

Toenail and Footcare Recipes

Toenail fungus and athlete's foot are common fungal infections that can be uncomfortable and unsightly. Nobody wants foot fungus. While multiple strategies may be needed to defeat a fungus, essential oils can support the body's natural defense against these infections and promote healthy skin and nails. Here are some essential oils for supporting the body in its fight against toenail fungus and Athlete's foot:

1. Tea Tree Oil (Melaleuca Alternifolia) - Tea tree oil has properties that may help protect against toenail fungus and athlete's foot. There is a study published in 2021 (https://pubmed.ncbi.nlm.nih.gov/33477259/) that shows Tea Tree works synergistically with medical treatment. Mix a few drops of tea tree oil with carrier oil, such as coconut oil, and apply to the affected area twice daily. I like to apply the oil and then put a bandage over it for a few hours to hold it in.

2. Red Cedar Bliss™ - A blend of oils that specifically supports skin, foot, and nail health. This would be a great blend to add to a spray bottle with a little witch hazel and make a foot spray. You could spay your feet as you get out of the shower each day for skin health support and prevention of fungal infections.

3. Oregano Oil - Oregano oil contains thymol and carvacrol, which have beneficial skin health properties. Mix a few drops of oregano oil with carrier oil and apply to the affected area twice daily.

4. <u>Lavender Oil</u> - Lavender oil has skin health and immune system supporting properties that can help feet and toenail health. Mix a few drops of Lavender oil with carrier oil and apply to the affected area twice daily.

5. <u>Eucalyptus Oil</u> - Eucalyptus foot skin and nail health-supporting properties. Mix a few drops of Eucalyptus oil with carrier oil and apply to the affected area twice daily.

6. <u>Lemongrass Oil</u> - Lemongrass oil has immune system-supporting properties and can help soothe irritated skin. Mix a few drops of Lemongrass oil with carrier oil and apply to the affected area twice daily.

7. <u>Peppermint Oil</u> - Peppermint oil has an immune system and skin-supporting properties and can help soothe itching and burning sensations. Mix a few drops of Peppermint oil with carrier oil and apply to the affected area twice daily.

8. <u>Egyptian Gold</u>™ - This blend of exotic oils supports clean, healthy skin and properties which discourage fungus. I have experience with this oil immediately taking the itch away from Athlete's foot.

Everyone responds differently to different oils. The above list you can try individually or blending several together to see what may work for you. Toenail fungus can be difficult to overcome, even when seeing a doctor. Even their prescribed antifungal internal medications don't always work. The best thing is to catch it early when it is just athlete's foot, before it spreads to toenails. You can also adopt a regimen of taking essential oils that are safe and approved for internal use in capsules to help the body fight in restoring balance against a fungus. Be prepared to battle for an extended period of time. And consult with your doctor or naturopath for their advice.

Chapter Eight

Summer Skin Care Recipes

Summer is a time to enjoy the sun, beach, and outdoor activities. However, our skin can also get exposed to harsh elements like sun, heat, and pollution. The good news is that essential oils can be a natural and effective way to protect, nourish, and revitalize your skin during summer. In this chapter, we will explore some of the best essential oils for summer skincare and provide easy-to-make recipes for after-sun spray, moisturizing lotion, and natural sunscreen.

Essential Oils for Summer Skincare

Lavender Essential Oil is well-known for its skin soothing and calming properties, making it perfect for after-sun care. It can also help to support the skin's natural inflammatory process and reduce redness caused by sunburn.

Peppermint Essential Oil has a cooling effect that can help to soothe sunburn and heat rash. It also has properties that can help to support the body in its fight against infection.

Tea Tree Essential Oil has many skin benefits and healthful properties. It can help to support the skin during acne breakouts, which can be exacerbated by sweat and heat during the summer.

Geranium Essential Oil is a natural astringent that can help to tighten and tone the skin. It can also help to balance oily or combination skin, which can be more prone to breakouts during the summer.

Recipe 1: **After-Sun Spray**

Ingredients:

- 1 cup distilled water

- 2 tablespoons aloe vera gel

- 10 drops of lavender essential oil

- 10 drops peppermint essential oil

Instructions:

1. In a small bowl, mix the aloe vera gel and essential oils.

2. Add the mixture to a spray bottle and fill it with distilled water.

3. Shake well before each use.

4. Spray onto the skin after sun exposure and gently rub in.

Recipe 2: **Moisturizing Lotion**

Ingredients:

- 1/2 cup coconut oil

- 1/4 cup sweet almond oil

- 1/4 cup shea butter

- 10 drops of geranium essential oil

Instructions:

1. In a double boiler, melt the coconut oil, sweet almond oil, and shea butter until thoroughly combined.
2. Remove from heat and let cool for 5 minutes.
3. Add the geranium essential oil and stir well.
4. Pour the mixture into a clean jar with a lid.
5. Let the lotion cool and solidify before using.
6. Apply to skin as needed for hydration and nourishment.

Recipe 3: **Natural Sunscreen**

Ingredients:

- 1/2 cup coconut oil

- 1/4 cup beeswax pellets

- 2 tablespoons zinc oxide powder

- 10 drops of lavender essential oil

- 10 drops of tea tree essential oil

Instructions:
1. Melt the coconut oil and beeswax pellets in a double boiler until thoroughly combined.
2. Remove from heat and let cool for 5 minutes.
3. Add the zinc oxide powder and essential oils and stir well.
4. Pour the mixture into a clean jar with a lid.
5. Let the sunscreen cool and solidify before using.

6. Apply to skin before sun exposure and reapply every 2 hours.

Recipe 4: **Natural Sunscreen #2**
Before Young Living came out with a clean and non-toxic 50 SPF sunscreen, I made this one every year.
Ingredients:

· ½ cup almond oil

· ½ cup liquid coconut oil

· ¼ cup beeswax pellets

· 2 TBSP zinc oxide

· 1 tsp red raspberry seed oil

· 2 TBSP shea butter

· 10 drops of lavender

· 10 drops of frankincense

Instructions:
1. Combine all the ingredients except zinc oxide in a pint-sized or larger glass jar.
2. Fill a medium saucepan with a couple of inches of water and place it on the stove over medium heat.
3. Put a lid loosely on the jar and place it in the pan with the water.
4. Shake or stir the jar occasionally to mix the ingredients as they melt.
5. When all the ingredients are completely melted, stir in the zinc oxide, and pour into whatever jar you use for storage.
6. Stir a few times as it cools to ensure zinc oxide is incorporated. Store at room temperature or in the refrigerator to increase shelf life.

Using essential oils in your summer skincare routine can benefit your skin. These recipes for after-sun spray, moisturizing lotion, and natural sunscreen are easy to make and can help to protect, nourish, and revitalize your skin during the summer months!

Chapter Nine

Fascia Care Recipes & Suggestions

Fascia is a connective tissue that surrounds and supports the body's muscles, bones, and organs. Proper fascia care is important for maintaining flexibility, mobility, and overall health. Physical Therapists recommend getting a massage every six weeks to help keep the fascia supple. Some people use massaging tools to work on their fascia at home. You can add essential oils with massage oil during a massage and daily to support fascia health and promote relaxation and relief from tension. Here are some natural essential oil remedies for fascia care:

1. Frankincense Oil - Frankincense oil has inflammatory support and discomfort-relieving properties that may help reduce tension and discomfort in the fascia. Apply a few drops of frankincense oil to the affected area with carrier oil and massage gently.

2. Peppermint Oil - Peppermint oil has cooling and soothing properties that can help relieve tension and discomfort in the fascia. Apply a few drops of peppermint oil to the affected area and massage gently. Use carrier oil if you prefer.

3. Ginger Oil - Ginger oil has warming and inflammatory support properties that may help reduce inflammation and discomfort in the fascia. Apply a few drops of ginger oil to the affected area and massage gently. Use carrier oil if you prefer.

4. Lavender Oil - Lavender oil has calming and relaxing properties that can help reduce tension and promote relaxation in the fascia. Apply a few drops of lavender oil to the affected area and massage gently. Use carrier oil if you prefer.

5. Rosemary Oil - Rosemary oil has stimulating and discomfort-relieving properties that may help relieve tension and discomfort in the fascia. Apply a few drops of rosemary oil and carrier oil (if preferred) to the affected area and massage gently.

Using natural essential oil remedies for fascia care can be a gentle and effective way to support overall health and well-being. If you have concerns about using essential oils for fascia care, consult a healthcare professional. Additionally, it is vital to maintain a healthy lifestyle, including regular exercise and stretching, to support fascia health.

Chapter Ten

Essential Oil Recipes for Heart Health

Essential oils naturally support heart health. Here are a few simple heart health recipes using essential oils:

1. Heart Health Smoothie

- 1 cup of frozen blueberries

- 1 banana

- 1/2 cup of unsweetened almond milk

- 1 tablespoon of chia seeds or Flax Hull Lignans

- 1 drop of Peppermint essential oil

Blend all ingredients until smooth. This smoothie may help support heart health by providing antioxidants and omega-3 fatty acids. (Flax Hull Lignans can be found at FlaxLignanHealth.com). I don't receive compensation for mentioning them; I've just used and loved this supplement for my family for years.

2. Blood Pressure-Reducing Diffuser Blend

- 3 drops of Lavender essential oil

- 3 drops of Ylang-ylang essential oil

- 3 drops of Frankincense essential oil

Add the essential oils to a diffuser and diffuse for 30 minutes. This blend supports normal blood pressure levels and promotes relaxation.

3. Healthy Cholesterol Salad Dressing

- 1/4 cup of extra-virgin olive oil

- 1 tablespoon of apple cider vinegar

- 1 teaspoon of honey

- 1/2 teaspoon of Dijon mustard

- 2 drops of lemon essential oil

Whisk all ingredients together and drizzle over a salad. This dressing may support healthy cholesterol levels and overall heart health.

4. Cardiovascular Support Massage Oil

- 1/4 cup of sweet Almond oil

- 5 drops of peppermint essential oil

- 5 drops of cypress essential oil

- 5 drops of rosemary essential oil

Mix the ingredients and massage into the chest and neck area. This massage oil may help support cardiovascular health and promote circulation.

Natural heart health recipes made with essential oils can help support heart health gently and naturally. If you have any heart condition or concerns, consult with your healthcare professional.

Chapter Eleven

Essential Oil Recipes for Respiratory Health

Essential oils can also be used to support respiratory health naturally. Here are a few simple respiratory health recipes using natural essential oils:

1. Congestion-Relieving Steam Inhalation

- 3 cups of boiling water

- 3 drops of eucalyptus essential oil – the variety called *Eucalyptus Globulus* smells just like Vicks™.

- 3 drops of peppermint essential oil

Add the essential oils to the boiling water and inhale the steam for 10-15 minutes. This steam inhalation may help relieve congestion and open the airways.

2. Respiratory Support Diffuser Blend

- 4 drops of eucalyptus or Raven™ essential oil

- 4 drops of tea tree essential oil

- 2 drops of lemon essential oil

Add the essential oils to a diffuser and diffuse for 30 minutes. This blend supports respiratory health and promotes a clear airway.

3. Seasonal Relief Rollerball

- 10 drops of lavender essential oil

- 10 drops of peppermint essential oil

- 10 drops of lemon essential oil

- 2 tablespoons of sweet almond oil or coconut

  oil

Mix the ingredients in a rollerball and apply to the chest and neck area. This rollerball may relieve sensitivities and seasonal discomforts and support respiratory health.

4. Cough-Relieving Chest Rub

- 1/4 cup of coconut oil

- 10 drops of eucalyptus or Raven™ essential oil

- 10 drops of peppermint essential oil

Mix the ingredients and apply to the chest and neck area. This chest rub may help relieve coughs and promote respiratory health.

5. Exercise-Induced Breathing Issue Roller Blend

- 10ml roller ball bottle

- 10 drops Idaho blue spruce oil

- 10 drops of peppermint oil

- 10 drops Raven™ oil

· Fill the rest of the roller ball bottle with coconut oil. Mix the ingredients and apply before, during, and after exercise to open the airways for easier breathing.

Natural respiratory health recipes made with essential oils can help gently and naturally support respiratory health.

Chapter Twelve

Essential Oil Recipes for Eye Health

Essential oils can be used to support eye health and improve vision. Here are some simple and natural essential oil remedies for eye health:

1. Eye Health Massage Blend

- 2 drops of lavender essential oil

- 2 drops of frankincense essential oil

- 2 tablespoons of sweet almond oil

Mix the ingredients together and gently massage around the eyes in a circular motion. This blend may help reduce eye strain, support healthy circulation, and promote relaxation. Also, drinking 4-6 oz a day of Ningxia Red (an antioxidant drink from Young Living that has lutein and zeaxanthin in it, nutrients for the eyes) is a great way to support your eye health.

2. Vision-Boosting Diffuser Blend

- 4 drops of cypress essential oil

- 4 drops of rosemary essential oil

- 2 drops of lemon essential oil

Add the essential oils to a diffuser and diffuse for 30 minutes. This blend may help your vision and support eye health.

3. Eye Soothing Compress

- 2 cups of warm water

- 2 drops of chamomile essential oil

- 2 drops of lavender essential oil

Soak a clean washcloth in the mixture and apply to closed eyes for 10-15 minutes. This compress may help soothe tired and dry eyes.

4. Dark Circle Reducing Serum

- 2 drops of rose essential oil

- 2 drops of sandalwood essential oil

- 1 tablespoon of jojoba oil

Mix the ingredients together and gently apply around the eyes. This serum may help reduce dark circles and puffiness around the eyes.

Using natural essential oil remedies for eye health can help promote healthy eyes and support healthy vision in a gentle and natural way. If you have any eye conditions or concerns, please speak with an eye specialist about using essential oils. Also, remember that if you get essential oils into your eyes and experience pain or discomfort, use a fatty carrier oil like coconut and wipe it into the eye, and then wipe it out. It will help relieve discomfort quickly.

Chapter Thirteen

Essential Oil Recipes for Brain Health

Essential oils can be used to support brain health and cognitive function. Here are some simple and natural essential oil remedies for brain health:

1. Brain Boosting Diffuser Blend

- 4 drops of peppermint essential oil

- 2 drops of lemon essential oil

Add the essential oils to a diffuser and diffuse for 30 minutes. This blend may help improve mental clarity and focus.

2. Memory-Boosting Roller Blend

- 2 drops of frankincense essential oil

- 2 drops of rosemary essential oil

- 2 drops of lemon essential oil

- 1 tablespoon of fractionated coconut oil

Mix the ingredients together and apply to the temples and back of the neck. This blend may help improve memory retention and cognitive function. I like to put blends like this in a 10ml roller ball bottle for easy use.

3. Stress-Reducing Inhaler Blend

- 4 drops of lavender essential oil
- 4 drops of Stress Away™ essential oil (or two drops of lime oil and 2 drops of vanilla oil)
- 4 drops of frankincense essential oil

Add the essential oils to an inhaler and inhale as needed. This blend may help reduce stress and promote relaxation.

4. Energizing Massage Blend

- 2 drops of peppermint essential oil
- 2 drops of rosemary essential oil
- 2 drops of lemon essential oil
- 2 tablespoons of sweet almond oil

Mix the ingredients together and gently massage onto the scalp and neck. This blend may help improve mental alertness and energy levels.

Young Living also has a blend called Clarity™ that is great to diffuse or roll under the nose. They also have a supplement *focus* drink called Ningxia Nitro that you can drink and get about 2-3 hours of good brain connectivity. I drink them before speaking in public, or if I need to concentrate to clean the garage or something that takes focus.

Using essential oils for brain health can help support healthy brain function and improve cognitive performance in a gentle and natural way. If you have any concerns about using essential oils for brain health, please consult with your naturopath or doctor before using.

Chapter Fourteen

Essential Oil Recipes for Hormone Support

Hormone imbalances can have a significant impact on overall health and well-being. Essential oils can be used to support hormone balance and promote a healthy endocrine system.

There is a product that Young Living has called Progessence Plus™. It is a natural progesterone essential oil serum that really is effective at balancing hormones, getting rid of menstrual cramping and relieving PMS and moodiness due to hormones. It also helps you to prevent miscarriages if you apply topically through at least the 14th week of pregnancy. I highly recommend that if you are a woman, you learn to incorporate this blend into your daily life.

Here is how you figure out your personal dose. Put 5-7 drops on the inside of your wrist and wait to see if your menstrual cramps, moodiness or achiness goes away within 15 minutes. If not, repeat the process. Do this every 15 minutes until the symptoms disappear. The total drops you needed is the dose your body wants. I need 5-7 drops but other people need 20+ drops. Your body is unique, you'll have to figure out your own dose.

Here are some other general natural essential oil remedies for hormone balancing that you can use:

1. Hormone Balancing Diffuser Blend

- 4 drops of clary sage essential oil

- 4 drops of lavender essential oil

- 2 drops of bergamot essential oil

Add the essential oils to a diffuser and diffuse for 30 minutes. This blend may help balance hormones and promote emotional well-being. Take the bergamot out and you have a deep-sleep diffuser blend that helps you get into a deep sleep and stay there most of the night.

2. Hormone Balancing Roller Blend

- 4 drops of clary sage essential oil

- 2 drops of frankincense essential oil

- 2 drops of ylang-ylang essential oil

- 1 tablespoon of fractionated coconut oil

Mix the ingredients together and apply to the wrists and back of the neck. This blend may help balance hormones and reduce symptoms of PMS.

3. Menopause Relief Bath Blend

- 2 drops of clary sage essential oil

- 2 drops of geranium essential oil

- 1 drop of lavender essential oil

- 1 cup of Epsom salt

Mix the essential oils with the Epsom salt and add to a warm bath. Soak for 20-30 minutes. This blend may help reduce symptoms of menopause and promote relaxation.

4. Fertility Boosting Massage Blend

- 2 drops of clary sage essential oil

- 2 drops of geranium essential oil

- 2 drops of bergamot essential oil

- 2 tablespoons of sweet almond oil

Mix the ingredients together and gently massage onto the lower abdomen. This blend may help support reproductive health and promote fertility.

Using natural essential oil remedies for hormone balancing can be a gentle and effective way to support overall health and well-being.

Chapter Fifteen

Essential Oil Recipes for Detoxification

Cleansing is an important aspect of maintaining overall health and well-being. Essential oils can be used to support the body's natural cleansing processes and promote a healthy immune system. Here are some natural essential oil remedies for cleansing:

1. Lemon Water Detox

- 1-2 drops of lemon essential oil

- 8 ounces of warm water

Mix the lemon essential oil with warm water and drink in the morning on an empty stomach. This blend may help support liver function and aid in digestion as well as help remove mucous from the cells.

2. Detoxifying Foot Soak

- 2 cups of Epsom salt

- 10 drops of peppermint essential oil

- 10 drops of lavender essential oil

Mix the Epsom salt and essential oils in a small tub of warm water and soak your feet for 20-30 minutes. This blend may help draw out toxins and promote relaxation.

3. Digestive Cleanse Roller Blend

- 8 drops of Ginger essential oil (or use the blend called Digize™)

- 12 drops of Peppermint essential oil

- fractionated coconut oil (about 10ml)

Mix the ingredients together and put in a 10ml roller ball bottle. and apply to the abdomen area. This blend may help promote healthy digestion and alleviate bloating.

4. Skin Detoxifying Mask

- 1 tablespoon of bentonite clay

- 1 drop of tea tree essential oil

- 1 drop of lavender essential oil

- 1 tablespoon of apple cider vinegar

Mix the bentonite clay, essential oils, and apple cider vinegar until smooth. Apply to the face and let dry for 10-15 minutes. Rinse with warm water. This blend may help draw out impurities and promote healthy skin.

Using essential oil remedies for cleansing can be a gentle and effective way to support overall health and well-being.

Chapter Sixteen

Essential Oil Recipes to Help with Weight Loss

Maintaining a healthy weight is important for overall health and well-being. While there is no magic solution for weight loss, incorporating natural essential oil remedies into your weight loss routine can be a helpful addition. Here are some natural essential oil remedies for weight loss:

1. Grapefruit Oil – Grapefruit oil has been shown to have properties that can aid in weight loss. It can help curb cravings and reduce appetite, making it easier to stick to a healthy diet. Add grapefruit oil to your water and drink daily. If it is a clean brand and labeled for internal use, take a capsule daily.

2. Lemon Oil - Lemon oil is known for its cleansing and detoxifying properties, which can aid in weight loss. It can help support digestion and boost metabolism. Add a drop of lemon oil (that is labeled for internal use) to a glass of water and drink it in the morning to help stimulate digestion and aid weight loss.

3. Peppermint Oil - Peppermint oil has been shown to have properties that can aid in weight loss. It can help reduce cravings and promote satiety, making it easier to stick to a healthy diet. Inhale peppermint oil directly from the bottle or diffuse it in a room to help reduce cravings.

4. <u>Cinnamon Oil</u> - Cinnamon oil has been shown to have properties that can aid in weight loss. It can help regulate blood sugar levels and boost metabolism. Add a drop of cinnamon oil (labeled for internal use) to your morning coffee or tea to help regulate blood sugar levels throughout the day.

5. <u>Citrus Fresh™ and Juva Cleanse™</u> are essential oils that you can combine with massage oil (or coconut oil) and apply to areas you want to reduce cellulite, detox, and possibly lose inches. You mix these oils and apply morning and night for 3 weeks. Take before and after pictures and measurements to see your progress.

6. <u>Cel-Lite™ Massage oil and Grapefruit oil</u> is another combination that you can put together to massage on your cellulite. Many people have reported that this reduces their cellulite.

7. <u>Ledum, Citrus Fresh™, and Grapefruit</u> - Add 15 drops of Ledum to a bottle of Citrus Fresh™ and put a roller ball on this bottle. Rub on your waist or whatever spot you want to reduce fat in at night and take a capsule of Grapefruit before bed. I did this for two weeks and lost 3 inches off my waist!

Using natural essential oil remedies for weight loss can be a helpful addition to a healthy diet and exercise routine. I have found that when I am actively trying to lose weight, and I use these protocols, I still need to try to get out and walk a mile or two a day – it just seems the weight comes off easier when I am using the essential oils. This is my personal experience. There is a theory that the citrus oils help strip mucous out of your cells. Mucous may provide a resistance to your cells releasing fat. So, if you can reduce the mucous, it is possible the fat can release better.

Additionally, it is important to maintain a healthy lifestyle, including regular exercise and a balanced diet, to support weight loss and overall health. Please consult with your doctor or naturopath about your own personal weight loss goals and what strategies to use.

Chapter Seventeen

Essential Oils That Relieve Discomfort

Living with pain can be a debilitating experience that can greatly affect your quality of life. While over-the-counter pain medications can provide temporary relief, they often come with negative side effects. Incorporating essential oils into your health routine can be a helpful addition. Here are some of the top natural essential oils that help with discomfort.

1. Peppermint Oil: Peppermint oil has a cooling and soothing effect that can provide support for the inflammatory process your body goes through when injured. You can apply peppermint around the hairline when you are experiencing headaches and migraines. The cooling sensation helps relax tension. Lay down in a cool, dark room with your eyes closed and relax. For other areas of the body, apply it directly to the affected area.

2. Clove Oil: Clove oil is known for its calming and soothing properties in the mouth. Dentists use it to numb gums. It can help alleviate tooth and gum discomfort. Mix a few drops of clove oil (labeled for internal use) with a carrier oil and apply it directly to the affected area.

3. Frankincense Oil: Frankincense oil has properties that can provide relief from discomfort. Mix equal drops with Idaho balsam fir oil, and copaiba oil and add to capsules to take internally. Try 3-4 capsules (about 28 drops total of each) for relief for severe discomfort like broken bones. I personally used this blend for 2 broken ribs and

was able to stick my fingers into my ribs and feel nothing! You may need a few more capsules if your body weight is on the higher end.

4. Idaho Balsam Fir: Idaho balsam fir oil has a fresh, clean aroma that can promote relaxation and ease muscle tension. It can help alleviate muscle and joint discomfort. Mix a few drops with a carrier oil and apply it directly to the affected area.

5. Copaiba: Copaiba oil has properties similar to CBD that can provide relief from discomfort. It can help alleviate muscle and joint discomfort and head discomfort. If it is approved for internal use, you can take this internally in capsules. For topical applications, mix a few drops of copaiba oil with a carrier oil and apply it directly to the affected area.

6. Valerian: Valerian oil is known for its sedative and discomfort-relieving properties. It can help alleviate muscle and joint discomfort as well as head discomfort. For topical applications, mix a few drops of Valerian oil with a carrier oil and apply it directly to the affected area.

7. Vetiver: Vetiver oil has a grounding and calming effect that can help alleviate discomfort caused by stress or tension. It can help alleviate muscle and joint discomfort. For topical applications, mix a few drops with a carrier oil and apply directly to the swollen or affected area.

8. Helichrysum: Helichrysum oil has properties that can provide relief from nerve discomfort. It also helps to support the regeneration of the nerves. It is cooling and supports a healthy inflammatory process. Mix a few drops of Helichrysum oil with a carrier oil and apply it directly to the affected area.

My favorite recipe that has helped people I know with *great discomfort* is:

- 5 drops Vetiver

- 10 drops Valerian

- 5 drops Helichrysum

- 2 drops Peppermint

Put these in a capsule. Take 1 capsule every 30 minutes until the discomfort goes away. You can take this for extreme discomfort, including after surgery.

One of my friends who struggles with MSA (Multiple Systems Atrophy) has struggled to find anything that gives her relief. She has spent many days and nights in incredible pain from her nerves and stomach. This recipe did it for her! She texted me, "That oil recipe took my pain to a ZERO!!!!! Nothing ever does that! I am so in awe and grateful and humbled!"

I know another person who used this remedy after a surgery to get pain relief.

Using essential oil remedies to relieve discomfort can be beneficial because the oils don't have side effects, don't make you loopy and aren't addictive.

Chapter Eighteen

Detox Bath Recipes

Detox baths can be a great way to unwind, relax and help eliminate toxins from the body. By adding essential oils to your bath, you can enhance the benefits and create a spa-like experience in the comfort of your own home. Here are ten different detox bath recipes that incorporate essential oils, with one recipe specifically designed for hormone balancing:

1. Lemon & Ginger Detox Bath

- 1 cup of Epsom salt

- 10 drops of lemon essential oil

- 5 drops of ginger or Digize™ essential oil

Add all ingredients to warm bathwater and soak for 20-30 minutes. This bath is great for improving digestion and boosting the immune system.

2. Lavender & Chamomile Relaxing Bath

- 1 cup of sea salt

- 10 drops of lavender essential oil

- 5 drops of chamomile essential oil

Add all ingredients to warm bathwater and soak for 20-30 minutes. This bath is great for promoting relaxation and reducing stress.

3. Lemon & Eucalyptus Sinus Relief Bath

- 1 cup of baking soda

- 10 drops of lemon essential oil

- 5 drops of eucalyptus essential oil

- 5 drops of peppermint on a rag (not in the bath)

Add all ingredients to warm bathwater and soak for 20-30 minutes. This bath is great for relieving sinus congestion and respiratory issues but beware that the peppermint will make you feel cold if you add it to the bath! Put 5 drops on a wet rag and hold it up to your nose to breathe in occasionally while soaking.

4. Exotic Rose & Ylang-Ylang Romantic Bath

- 1 cup of Himalayan pink salt

- 10 drops of rose essential oil (or substitute jasmine)

- 5 drops of ylang-ylang essential oil

Add all ingredients to warm bathwater and soak for 20-30 minutes. This bath is great for promoting love and romance. A good rose oil is extremely pricey, this is definitely a special occasion bath!

5. Tea Tree & Lavender Soothing Bath

- 1 cup of sea salt

- 10 drops of tea tree essential oil

- 5 drops of lavender essential oil

Add all ingredients to warm bathwater and soak for 20-30 minutes. This bath is great for soothing irritated skin and supporting your body's inflammatory process.

6. Orange & Vanilla Calming Bath

- 1 cup of Epsom salt

- 10 drops of orange essential oil

- 5 drops of vanilla essential oil

- Add all ingredients to warm bathwater and soak for 20-30 minutes. This bath is great for calming the mind and reducing anxiety. Beware that orange oil is photosensitive, so this is not good to do the night before spending a day in the sun.

7. Frankincense & Myrrh Anti-Aging Bath

- 1 cup of sea salt

- 10 drops of frankincense essential oil

- 5 drops of myrrh essential oil

Add all ingredients to warm bathwater and soak for 20-30 minutes. This bath is great for reducing the appearance of fine lines and wrinkles.

8. Grapefruit & Juniper Detox Bath

- 1 cup of sea salt

- 10 drops of grapefruit essential oil

- 5 drops of juniper essential oil

Add all ingredients to warm bathwater and soak for 20-30 minutes. This bath is great for eliminating toxins and reducing fluid retention. Beware of photosensitivity. Don't use this bath combination if you are going out in the sun the next day.

9. Hormone Balancing Bath

- 1 cup of Epsom salt

- 10 drops of clary sage essential oil

- 5 drops of Idaho balsam fir essential oil

- 5 drops of copaiba essential oil

- Add all ingredients to warm bathwater and soak for 20-30 minutes. This bath is great for balancing hormones and reducing symptoms of PMS.

10. Muscle-Soothing Bath

- 1 cup Epsom salt

- 1/2 cup baking soda

- 10 drops copaiba essential oil

- 10 drops lavender essential oil

- 5 drops eucalyptus essential oil

Instructions:

1. Fill the bathtub with warm water.

2. Add 1 cup of Epsom salt and 1/2 cup of baking soda to the water and stir until dissolved.

3. Add essential oils to the water and mix well.

4. Soak in the bath for 20-30 minutes to allow the oils to penetrate your muscles and relax tension.

5. After soaking, rinse off with warm water and pat dry with a towel.

Chapter Nineteen

Kids Roller Blend Recipes

Essential oils can be a great support to your child's health and wellness regimen. One easy and convenient way to use them for kids is by creating roller blends. Roller blends are a diluted mixture of essential oils that can be applied directly to the skin using a rollerball applicator. Kids love to have their own roller ball bottles that are diluted and ready to go. These recipes are all figured for a 10ml roller ball bottle which you can get online at various retailers. Here are some essential oil recipes for kids' roller blends:

1. Immune Support Roller Blend

- 15 drops Thieves™ essential oil

- 5 drops lemon essential oil

- 5 drops frankincense essential oil

- 10 ml fractionated coconut oil

Directions: Combine the essential oils and Fractionated Coconut Oil in a rollerball bottle. Roll onto the bottoms of your child's feet and along their spine to support their immune system.

2. Calming Roller Blend

- 10 drops lavender essential oil

- 15 drops Peace and Calming™ essential oil

- 10 ml Fractionated Coconut Oil

Directions: Combine the essential oils and Fractionated Coconut Oil in a rollerball bottle. Roll onto your child's wrists, behind their ears, and on the bottoms of their feet to promote feelings of calm and relaxation.

3. Focus and Concentration Roller Blend

- 10 drops peppermint essential oil

- 10 drops rosemary essential oil

- 5 drops lemon essential oil

- 10 ml fractionated coconut oil

Directions: Combine the essential oils and Fractionated Coconut Oil in a rollerball bottle. Roll onto your child's temples, back of the neck, and wrists to improve their focus and concentration.

4. Sleep Support Roller Blend

- 10 drops lavender essential oil

- 10 drops cedarwood essential oil

- 5 drops vetiver essential oil

- 10 ml fractionated coconut oil

Directions: Combine the essential oils and Fractionated Coconut Oil in a rollerball bottle. Roll onto the bottoms of your child's feet and along their spine before bed to promote a restful night's sleep.

5. Tummy Helper Roller Blend

- 10 drops DiGize™ essential oil (or use ginger and fennel essential oil)

- 10 drops peppermint essential oil

- 10 ml fractionated coconut oil

Directions: Combine the essential oils and fractionated coconut oil in a rollerball bottle. Roll onto your child's tummy in a clockwise motion to help ease stomach discomfort.

Note: Always make sure to use high-quality essential oils that have been distilled in surgical stainless steel. You don't want aluminum toxicity in your child's oils! Young Living is the brand I recommend for safety!

Chapter Twenty

Autoimmune Support Recipes

Autoimmune diseases occur when the immune system mistakenly attacks healthy cells and tissues in the body. Symptoms of autoimmune diseases can vary depending on the type of disease and the affected area. While essential oils are not a cure for autoimmune diseases, they may provide support for the immune system and help manage some symptoms.

1. **Frankincense Roller Blend:** Frankincense has properties that can help support the body's immune system as well as it's inflammatory response. This roller blend can be applied to the back of the neck, wrists, and soles of the feet to promote relaxation and balance.

- 10 drops frankincense essential oil

- 10 drops lavender essential oil

- 5 drops peppermint essential oil

- 10 ml fractionated coconut oil

Add all ingredients to a roller bottle and shake well before use.

2. **Immune Support Roller Blend:** This is a natural immune system support blend. This blend can be

applied to the chest, back of the neck, and wrists to provide immune support.

- 10 drops lemon essential oil

- 10 drops peppermint essential oil

- 10 drops frankincense essential oil

- 10 ml fractionated coconut oil

Add all ingredients to a roller bottle and shake well before use.

3. **Auto-Immune Support Roller Blend**: This blend can be applied to the affected area to provide relief and inflammatory system support.

- 10 drops oregano oil

- 10 drops basil essential oil

- 10 drops rosemary essential oil

- 10 drops thyme essential oil

- 10 drops cypress essential oil

- 10 drops Valor™ essential oil

- 10 ml fractionated coconut oil

Add all ingredients to a roller bottle and shake well before use.

Add all ingredients to a roller bottle or container and shake well before use. You can use the entire bottle on the spine and rub in if you like in one sitting. This is not a replacement for but is similar in theory to the Raindrop oils. The Raindrop Massage is something many people with auto-immune issues get relief from. I have a podcast about the Raindrop Massage you can listen to. The podcast is called "The Oily Academy" and it is on most all major podcast apps like Apple Podcasts and Spotify. It is episode 95 and is called, "The Raindrop Technique As Your Family Power Tool."

4. **Digestive Support Roller Blend:** Autoimmune diseases can often affect the digestive system. This blend can be applied to the abdomen to support digestion and reduce discomfort.

- 10 drops peppermint essential oil

- 15 drops DiGize™

- 10 ml fractionated coconut oil

Add all ingredients to a roller bottle and shake well before use.

5. **Hormone Balancing Roller Blend**: Autoimmune diseases can disrupt the endocrine system and cause hormone imbalances. This blend can be applied to the lower abdomen and lower back to support hormone balance.

- 10 drops clary sage essential oil

- 10 drops geranium essential oil

- 5 drops ylang-ylang essential oil

- (Optional powerful addition: 20 drops Progessence Plus™)

- 9 ml fractionated coconut oil

Add all ingredients to a roller bottle and shake well before use.

6. **Stress Relief Roller Blend**: Autoimmune diseases can cause stress and anxiety. This blend can be applied to the wrists and behind the ears to promote relaxation and reduce stress.

- 10 drops lavender essential oil

- 10 drops bergamot essential oil

- 5 drops frankincense essential oil

- 10 ml fractionated coconut oil

Add all ingredients to a roller bottle and shake well before use.

7. **Discomfort Roller Blend**: This blend can be applied to the affected area to reduce discomfort and support your body's inflammatory response.

- 10 drops peppermint essential oil

- 10 drops PanAway™ essential oil

- 10 drops frankincense essential oil

- 10 ml fractionated coconut oil

Add all ingredients to a roller bottle and shake well before use.

8. **Respiratory Support Roller Blend**: This blend can be applied to the chest and back to support respiratory function.

- 10 drops Raven™ or a eucalyptus variety essential oil

- 10 drops peppermint essential oil

- 10 drops lemon essential oil

- 10 ml fractionated coconut oil

Add all ingredients to a roller bottle and shake well before use.

Chapter Twenty-One

Conclusion

As more and more people become aware of the potential risks and side effects associated with conventional drugs and chemical-based home products, the demand for natural health remedies and alternatives has continued to grow.

Really, it is with good reason. Pure, clean essential oils that have been distilled properly offer a safe and effective way to promote overall health and wellness without the potentially harmful side effects associated with many conventional products.

Thank you for allowing me to share my love of essential oils, and some of the recipes I know and love with you. I have been using essential oils for twenty years and believe they have kept my family healthier and out of the doctor's office most of the time.

Essential oils offer a powerful and effective way to support our health naturally. With the right brand of oils and proper usage, you can feel safe and confident in using essential oils to support your health and well-being.

If you are looking for a good place to buy your oils, I recommend checking out YoungLiving.com. They have been in business for almost 30 years and were the pioneers in bringing essential oils to the United States. Many other companies have come along since and jumped on the essential oil bandwagon, but Young Living sets the standards.

Young Living is much like Costco or Sam's Club. You make an initial purchase of 100pv ($100) and that qualifies you for a one-year membership where you get 24% off the retail prices. You are always welcome to buy one oil or have your total under $100, you just have to pay retail pricing. Also, when you become a member, you are not a distributor or a reseller. Unlike some multi-level marketing companies that "sign you up" and automatically treat you like you are a distributor, Young Living has 95% of members who are only customers. There is no pressure for you to sell anything. You are a customer. If you are interested in becoming a reseller, it takes extra steps, and I can help you with that.

If you are interested in purchasing from Young Living and would like my expertise in helping you learn more about essential oils, and my customer service support, use my enroller/sponsor number (#1062622) when you check out. I'd love to have you on my team. Thank you for supporting small businesses and helping this mom of three boys work from home.

And if instead you have found your own favorite brand of essential oils and know they are distilled correctly and you feel safe using them, *thank you still for reading my book and for using natural health to support your family.* Us natural health lovers need to stick together. I wish every reader to find their way to natural health and wellness!

About Wendy Selvig

I am a Certified Aromatherapist.

Here is a photo of my certificate:

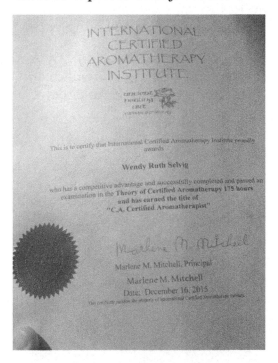

I am also Certified in the Raindrop Technique and am a C.R.T.S (Certified Raindrop Technique Specialist). The Raindrop Technique is a special massage-like technique that uses essential oils. It is a wonderful and powerful tool to use any time your immune system needs support, or if you have an auto-immune disease you are fighting against.

My friend Amber Grady (who is also a CRTS) and I wrote a book called, *The Power of a Raindrop* for the average person to learn how to give them and to not feel overwhelmed with the process. The Raindrop is what I call the "Natural Health Power Tool" and is what we pull out for our family if there is any kind of scary diagnosis or serious issue where your body needs support. However, once you start giving Raindrops to your significant other and children, you'll find it is a special connection where you can use the power of touch to apply the oils. Your family will love it and it is a tool to connect emotionally and give loving care to your loved ones. The Raindrop oils all come in a kit and are available at YoungLiving.com.

The book, *The Power of A Raindrop,* by Amber Grady and Wendy Selvig is available at GrowingHealthyHomes.com.

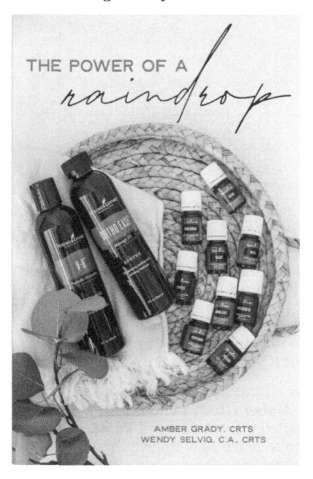

THE POWER OF A *raindrop*

AMBER GRADY. CRTS
WENDY SELVIG. C.A.. CRTS

WAYS TO FIND ME:

TheOilyAcademy.com

The Oily Academy Podcast

Info@theoilyacademy.com

Multiple books for sale on Amazon, search for author
Wendy Selvig.

YoungLiving.Com – Join and use enroller #1062622 to
be assigned to my team.

Interested in Natural Health?

TAKE A QUIZ & CONNECT WITH ME & FIND OUT WHAT YL PRODUCTS WILL HELP YOU PERSONALLY!

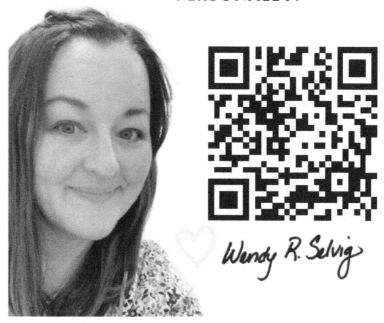

Wendy R. Selvig

Scan this code with your smartphone and it will take you to a Google form I have made where you can get in touch with me directly! You can tell me about some of your health goals and I'll tell you (based on being in the company since 2008 and knowing the products really well) which oils and supplements will help you accomplish your goals. The quiz is free and there is no obligation to buy anything. Knowledge is power! Connect with me!

Want to look into selling Young Living oils and supplements yourself?

Contact me. If you are a business minded person, I'd love to talk to you. Send me an email at info@thoilyacademy.com.

After years of sticking with it and trying different methods, I have found a way to sustainably build my business over time, slowly. (Hint: It is not by writing books.) ☺ I have been able to build my business to gold level with Young Living which brings in enough income for me to stay home with my kids. You can search the internet for "Young Living Income Disclosure Statement" to see how much that might be.

If you want to team up with me, I will show you how. Multi-level marketing is tricky, and I despise traditional methods of trying to get all your friends and family involved. My method involves leaving out your friends and family (unless they ask, of course.). You can't build a business off your friends and family anyway; you eventually have to be successful in circles outside of yourself. So, let's just start there to begin with. It takes the pressure off, and you can build and grow your business without feeling like you have pressured anyone inside your inner circle.

Want to know more? Shoot me an email!

The End.

Made in United States
Orlando, FL
26 April 2023